# Student Nurse Ward Basics

Learn the basics of everything and get ward ready in a flash!

# Student Nurse Ward Basics

David Wills
RGN

Published by
HIGHINSPIRE PUBLISHING

# HIGHINSPIRE

First published   2017

# CONTENTS

Being a Student.................................................................7

Common Medication..........................................................9

Complaints and Procedures.............................................26

Essential Anatomy and Physiology.................................43

Abbreviations..................................................................49

Administrations Route.....................................................54

Communication................................................................55

Patient Communication...................................................58

Index...............................................................................60

# Student Nurse Ward Basics
# (LEARNING MADE EASY)

## Preface

The ESSENTIAL student nurse ward basics is an easy to read book that takes the student nurse through all the basic essentials they need to know about working within the hospital. David Wills is a registered general nurse with over 23 years healthcare experience and feels that it's time to learn the basics via the simplest method and will guide you through everything you need to know before starting work within a hospital ward.

This will give you a serious head start and will put you way out in front of your colleagues when it comes to drug, ward and medical knowledge. They will be amazed at what you know and how quick you are learning.

Below is a list of essentials you will easily be able to master within two weeks.

The course will take the student nurse through the:

•        Most common drugs that are used within a hospital.

•        Most common medical complaints.

•        Essential anatomy and physiology.

•        Common abbreviations.

•        Communication.

•        Life as a student nurse.

# ACKNOWLEDGMENTS

To Minnie, I'm very proud of your achievements.
Maria and Ricky, Remembering you always.

# BEING A STUDENT

So, you are a student once again, studying a subject that is as vast as the eye can see. Being a student nurse is like learning to drive!.... (You get tested on a million and one scenarios and subjects but when you pass your test it's all about driving to the speed limit and avoiding the other cars.)

For me, it's quite the same with nursing. Throughout ones' training, I was taught a wide variety of knowledge, such as government statistics and polices, models of nursing, standards of practice that seem like they were from the dark ages. It always left me thinking, is this really going to be necessary when I start work after my nursing hand over? For me, the answer was no, it was not necessary. The three pharmacology lessons I received during my three years training were not nearly enough to teach me the contents of my drug cabinet during my morning medication round.

There is great deal to learn about nursing, patient care and bed side manner, but I also feel that certain people teaching nursing courses are somewhat detached and unaware of ward work routine.

Just like going back to the driving test, it's like learning the inner workings of a car and the philosophy behind the early transport system before even knowing what the clutch is for!

I feel that everything should start from the basics and not be taught via the hardest method just because it can be.

Whilst working within the hospital, the student nurse will come across the same words, drugs, phrases, abbreviations, jargon and procedures across the board.

You may very well hear things like: Patient has IDC but TWOC AM tomorrow after CT then 20mg of reg Furosemide BD, STAT anti emetic and PRN Oramorph and metaclopramide. You may very well be left thinking that all those hours of studying government polices from 1972 has prepared you for what you have just heard!

As hand over continues at a fast pace with a multitude of jargon and abbreviations, it is over before you know it and are given some patients to look after. You think to yourself, what is BD and IDC (do other wards use this?), what is Metaclopramide, (is this a common drug or specialist drug?)

It would be so much easier having a good understanding of basic grass roots knowledge of common drugs, procedures and abbreviations.

There are certain drugs that most adult patients will be taking on a day to day basis. These will be drugs like aspirin, beta blockers and Senna (laxatives).

These are very interesting drugs to start learning about as patients often ask what their tablets are for.

The first chapter of the book will look at the most used common medication that are used within a hospital setting.

After listening to the CD, cover up the description of titled drug and give your own description of what you think the drug is. The more you do this, the more you will recognise drugs and be able to give you own drug descriptions.

Around 80% of all patients will be on some sort of pain relief, so the first part of the next chapter will look at common pain killers and analgesic medication.

Let's go!

# COMMON MEDICATIONS
## Pain Relief (Ouch!!)

## Co-codamol
## Pain, inflammation and high temperature

This belongs to the group of medicines known as analgesics.

Co-codamol contains a combination of two pain-killing ingredients paracetamol and codeine. It is used to stop pain and reduce inflammation and fever (high temperature).

Co-codamol can be used to relieve pain and inflammation caused by rheumatic and muscular pain, sprains, strains, backache, headache, sore throat, toothache and period pain. It is also useful in treating cold and 'flu-like' symptoms and reducing fever (high temperature).

Co-codamol is available in tablet, capsule and soluble tablet form.
Tip 1: your Co-codamol box may also say Kapake; KapakeInsts; Medocodene; Migraleve; Paracodol; Parake; Solpadol or Tylex. These are different manufacturers versions of this drug. They should all have the same desired affect but come from different suppliers/drug companies.

Tip 2: if there is no strength written on the drug chart and you really need to give the medication, give the lower dose and get the prescribing doctor to write up the desired strength.

## Paracetamol
## Pain and high temperature (pyrexia)

Paracetamol can be used to relieve mild to moderate aches and pains associated with conditions such as headaches, migraine, toothache, teething, colds and flu. It is also useful for reducing fever and discomfort associated with colds and flu and following vaccinations.

Tip 1: be aware that many drugs contain paracetamol, such as Co-codamol. It is a well-known and common mistake to overdose the patient on too much paracetamol due to paracetamol and Co-codamol written on the same drug/prescription chart.

Tip 2: check STAT (once only) and PRN (as and when required) part of the drug /prescription chart for Co-codamol or any other drug that contains paracetamol, and if found tell the nurse in charge, pharmacy and/or doctors and then give yourself a pat on the back for double checking.

## Ibuprofen

## Pain tenderness inflammation (swelling) stiffness

Ibuprofen is used to relieve the pain, tenderness, inflammation (swelling), and stiffness caused by arthritis and gout. It is also used to reduce fever and to relieve headaches, muscle aches, menstrual pain, aches and pains from the common cold, backache, and pain after surgery or dental work.

## Aspirin

## Mild and moderate pain

Aspirin is used to relieve mild to moderate pain; reduce fever, redness, and swelling. This will usually be dissolved in water and given in 75mg or 150mg. Aspirin also has some blood thinning properties and may well be given to thin the patient's blood.

The last three pain relief medication. are to treat mild to moderate pain.

## CD

The abbreviation CD stands for **controlled drug**. This means that there are extra protocols a nurse should abide by when administering controlled drugs so ensure you check with your line manager or mentor before handling CD's.

Tip: Controlled drugs must also be discarded in a particular way so (again) check with your mentor or line manager before discarding such drugs.

Stop, think, and protect your pin!

## Dihydrocodeine (CD)

## Moderate to severe pain

Dihydrocodeine tartrate belongs to a group of medicines called opioids. Opioids mimic the effects of naturally occurring pain reducing chemicals (endorphins). They combine with the opioid receptors in the brain and block the transmission of pain signals. Therefore, even though the cause of the pain may remain, less pain is actually felt. Can be given in either form tablet or injection

Tip: this medication should be taken with food.

## Oxycodine (CD) (hydrochloride) CD

## Moderate to severe pain.

Opioid based oral medication. Patients with cancer and with post operative pain.

## Morphine (CD)

## Severe pain

Morphine is used to relieve moderate to severe pain. Morphine is in a class of medications called opioid analgesics. It works by affecting the way the body senses pain. Morphine is generally given in three different formats: Oral(Oramorph)(MST), IM (intramuscular injection). or IV (pump).

## Oramorph SR (CD) **(sustained release)**

### Severe pain reliever

Relieves moderate to severe pain. Morphine may also be used to treat pain associated with cancer, heart attacks, sickle cell disease and other medical conditions. This type of morphine is for people who need pain medicine for more than a few days. These capsules and tablets are especially designed to release morphine over a period of time

Each **Oramorph** SR Tablet contains 15 mg, 30 mg, 60 mg, or 100 mg morphine sulphate. Sustained release means that this drug releases its effect slowly in to the body and acting over longer periods

## Morphine injection

### Fast acting break thorough pain

When injected intravenously, morphine can produce intense euphoria and a general state of well-being and relaxation. Regular use can result in the rapid development of tolerance to these effects also known as dependence.

## Morphine pump

### Prolonged pain relief

This method of controlling morphine application is by fitting an external pump that will be under the patient's control. This administers doses into the body as needed and is set up before hand according to the doctors' regime. Also known as patient controlled administration (PCA).

Opioid based medication also comes as a patch. This patch is called Fentanyl and usually is applied to the patients arm. This is good for patients that are having difficulty in swallowing (dysphagia).

Antiemetic Drugs (Anti sickness)

# Metoclopramide

## **Antiemetic/Anti sickness**

Metoclopramide (Maxilon) is a medicine that increases the movements or contractions of the stomach and intestines. When given by injection, it is used to help diagnose certain problems of the stomach and/or intestines. It is also used by injection to prevent the nausea and vomiting that may occur after treatment with anticancer medicines. Another medicine may be used with Metoclopramide to prevent side effects that may occur when Metoclopramide is used with anticancer medicines.

# Cyclizine **(Prochlorperazine)**

## **Nausea and Vomiting**

Cyclizine is used to relieve nausea, vomiting, and dizziness associated with motion sickness. Can be given in tablet form or as an injection. Cyclizine is usually the preferred injection following Morphine medication.

# Prochlorperazine

## **Antiemetic/anti sickness**

Prochlorperazine is an oral and parenteral antiemetic and antipsychotic drug. Usually given for motion sickness, vertigo and nausea.

# Heart Medication/Cardiac drugs

## Atenolol

## Blood pressure/Beta-blocker

Used for lowering heart rate and lowering blood pressure. Atenolol blocks the action of the sympathetic nervous system, a portion of the involuntary nervous system. The sympathetic nervous system stimulates the pace of the heart beat. By blocking the action of these nerves, atenolol reduces the heart rate and is useful in treating abnormally rapid heart rhythms. Atenolol also reduces the force of heart muscle contraction and lowers blood pressure.

## Digoxin

## Heart failure

Digoxin will assist the heart towards having a regular heart beat and rhythm rather than an irregular one. It is also used to treat hear failure.

## Amlodipine

## High blood pressure and chest pain

This drug is called a calcium channel blocker/ACE inhibitor and can be used for treating high blood pressure and chest pain (angina).

## Bendroflumethiazide (formerly bendrofluazide)

## Hypertension (high blood pressure)

Also, called water, fluid tablets or diuretics, works by increasing the amount of urine patients produce.

## Amiodarone

### Irregular heartbeats

Amiodarone is used to help keep the heart beating normally in people with life-threatening heart rhythm disorders.

## Atorvastatin

### Heart attack prevention

Used to reduce and slow the amount of cholesterol and fat intake within the blood and will help prevent the heart and blood vessels from clogging up with fatty deposits.

## Ramipril

### High blood pressure and heart failure

Ramipril (Altace) is an ACE inhibitor. (angiotensin converting enzyme). Ramipril is used to treat high blood pressure (hypertension) and congestive heart failure. This drug is sometimes given to patients following a heart attack.

## Lansoprazole

### Gastric and duodenal ulcers

Prevents the production of acid in the stomach. It reduces symptoms and prevents injury to the oesophagus or stomach in patients with gastroesophageal reflux disease (GORD) or ulcers.

## Ranitidine

### Reduce gastric acid

This drug helps reduce gastric acidity and prevents ulcers from coming back.

Omeprazole

## Stomach pain and ulcers

Reduces and blocks the production of stomach acids, and prevents pain and ulcers.

**Sleeping Tablets**

Zopiclone

## Trouble in sleeping

This drug is used to treat insomnia and for people that are having difficulty in sleeping. They act on the central nervous system and should only be used for short periods of time.

Diazepam

## Insomnia and alcohol withdrawal

This drug is used to treat short term anxiety or insomnia/sleeping difficulties when alcohol withdrawal is taking place.

Haloperidol

## Violent, dangerous and impulsive behaviour

This drug is used to calm patients down, making them less anxious and will also help them to sleep.

**Breathing**

Nebulizers

# Airway and Breathing

A nebulizer is any machine that uses compressed air to turn liquid in to a fine mist that can be inhaled by the patient. This usually is a small electrically powered box that allows a single air hose to be attached to it. There are different types of solutions the patient could be receiving, depending on the particular type of breathing complaint.

## Salbutamol

## Asthma and Airway obstruction

This is a beta2 agonist and bronchodilator, used to relax and widen the patient's airways so that they can breathe more easily.

## Atrovent  (Ipratropium bromide)

## Breathing and prevent bronchospasm.

This drug used to relax and to prevent bronchospasm in the airway.

## Combivent

## Widening of the airway/bronchodilator

Relaxes muscles in the airways, and improves the patients breathing.

## Pulmicort

## Breathing and airway

Pulmicort is a steroid base anti-inflammatory nebulizer to maintain the patency of the patient's airway and to help them breathe.
It is not a fast acting medication and is used for preventative measures.

## Inhalers

### **Breathing and airway**

Inhalers are for patients that self medicate with most of the above nebulizers to help them breathe better. Sometime these can be called puffers and can (in some cases) have an air chamber that can be attached to them for the patient to receive the full dose for medication required.

## Antibiotics

Antibiotics kill bacteria that has entered in to and lives within the body. These bacteria are single-cell organisms. When bacteria pass our immune systems and start reproducing inside the bodies, they cause disease. Antibiotics will work to kill the bacteria to eliminate this disease.

Bacteria can also stop or prevent certain parts of the body from working by sometimes producing harmful chemicals.

### **Prophylactic**
means that a drug or antibiotic is used in defence or as prevention. In other words, "Just in case the patient gets an infection"

## Erythromycin

### **Fight infection. Tonsillitis, bronchitis, pneumonia, whooping cough, Legionnaire's disease, chlamydia, gonorrhoea, skin infections, and other infections.**

This very commonly used antibiotic is used to treat bacterial infections within the body and throat and chest infections.

## Clarithromycin

### Tonsillitis, bronchitis, pneumonia, whooping cough, Legionnaire's disease, Chlamydia, gonorrhoea, skin infections, and other infections.

Clarithromycin is a semi-synthetic derivative of erythromycin and is sometimes used for patients that are intolerant of erythromycin.

## Amoxicillin

### Pneumonia, bronchitis, gonorrhoea, ear infections, nose, throat, urinary tract, skin infections and others. It is also used in combination with other medications.

This commonly used antibiotic is used bacterial infections.
Mostly given in tablet form but can also be given IV (intra Venous in the vein via a drip)

Tip: Antibiotics are always given as a course. This means that the whole course, box or bottle of antibiotics must be taken (Not all at once), even if the patient feels better and feels that he or she does not need them anymore. By not taking antibiotics properly this can result in bacteria growing resistant and therefore making some antibiotics having little or no effect.

## Penicillin

### Kills bacteria Tonsillitis, pneumonia, strep throat, bronchitis, and infections of the skin.

This is yet another and probably the most commonly known antibiotic of all and is used to fight infection within the body. This particular antibiotic can sometime be used in conjunction with other antibiotics, such as Amoxicillin.

## Vancomycin

### <u>Antibiotic, Fight infection.</u>

Vancomycin is an IV antibiotic but can also be given to the patient orally. It is used to treat infections were sometimes other antibiotics have failed. It can be used for infections such as gram-positive cocci or Staphylococcus aurous and for the more serious infections.

This medication (along with other medication) causes side effects and could cause damage to hearing and kidneys. The nurse will usually have to make this medication up by diluting vials of Vancomycin powder with water/saline and adding this to a mini-bag (small bag of fluid).

A basic IV (intra venous) separate course (CPD = Continued Professional Development) needs to be undertaken before a qualified nurse is able to deal with IV medication and drug additives.

Tip 1: Ask your line manager will know about IV courses.

Tip 2: At some point, the patient will need to be checked by the doctor to see how much Vancomycin is in the patient's body. This is called "Vanc levels". The doctor should come around every few days and check for Vanc levels on patients that are in receipt of Vancomycin.

## Metronidazole

### <u>Antibiotic. Fights bacteria.</u>

This medication is good for treating conditions such as acne, colitis and other dermatological (skin) infections. Metronidazole is an anaerobic antibiotic (antibiotics that are able to grow without oxygen). You will sometimes see this antibiotic being used with Cefuroxime.

# Cefuroxime

## **Bacteria infections, such as bronchitis; gonorrhoea; Lyme disease; and infections of the ears, throat, sinuses, urinary tract, and skin.**

Can be given in IV or in tablet form. Also works in conjunction with Metronidazole.

Tip: If the patient is written up for Cefuroxime or Metronidazole, check and see if there are any readymade bags in the drugs fridge. Or if time is a factor, find out if the pharmacy or sterile department can make some up for the patient.

# Gentamicin

## **Eye and skin infections**

This type of antibiotic is used to treat infections that are made up of many different types of bacteria. This is usually given via IV or injection.

# AUGMENTIN

## **Broad spectrum antibiotic, to fight infection**

Also known as (Co-amoxiclav), this antibiotic is able tackle a very wide range of infections. This is sometimes used when doctors are not sure of the cause of the origin of the infection and is sometimes used when a patient's infection is not fully understood.

## Miscellaneous drugs

These are drugs that are still very popular and are used throughout the hospital.

## Ferrous Sulphate

## Forming red blood cells and oxygen storage

Ferrous sulphate is an iron preparation. Iron is a vital component of haemoglobin (oxygen-carrying pigment of red blood cells.)

Tip: In some cases, iron, may make the patients stool discoloured and dark. The patient may worry about this in the first instance.

## THYROXINE (Hormone)

## Hypothyroidism (under active thyroid gland)

This is usually a treatment for patients that have an under active thyroid gland and need some replacement therapy, this therapy come in the form of Thyroxine.

## Insulin

## Regulation of blood sugar for type one diabetics only

Insulin is a natural hormone that regulates blood glucose levels within the body. People with type one diabetes need to have injections of insulin to control the amount of glucose in their bloodstream. Insulin injections act as a replacement for natural insulin and allow people with diabetes to achieve normal blood glucose levels.

There are different types of insulin available on the ward and the modern day method of giving this sort of medication is via a pen. The patient can be easily educated on how to use the pen and will therefore give the patient more opportunity to self medicate when it is time for discharge. There is also less room for drug errors as most of the pens on the market have a dial that is easily turned to the amount of units that is prescribed for the patient, making it clearer

and easier to give the correct amount of insulin. Some pens use replaceable cartridges of insulin and other models are disposable.

Some patients need intense regulation of their insulin levels, these patients maybe on a sliding scale insulin pump. This will be a small infusion pump that will deliver a precise amount of insulin every hour depending on the amount of sugar the patient has in their blood.

The nurse will take the level of sugar via a glucometer (small blood sugar testing machine) and adjust the pump accordingly. The ratio will be written by the doctor on the patients' prescription/drug chart.

Tip: Some hospitals require nurses to be IV trained before setting rates on infusion pumps. Take great care with infusion pumps and check before you go pushing any buttons (even the stop and start button). Infusion pumps are renowned for occluding (Blocking) and alarming. If this happens, check with the line manager before doing anything (some are stricter than others and one may say **yes** while the other one may say **no**.

## Insulin jet injectors

## <u>Insulin injection without the needle</u>

These send a fine spray of insulin through the skin by a high-pressure air mechanism instead of needles. These are great for people, who fear needles, but they're expensive and you have to sterilize the units frequently.

This is a very new and modern day way of giving medication. You may have seen medication being giving this way in the programme *Star Trek*. Trials are still going on with this method and we may well see more and more medication being given like this.

Some of the different typed for insulin include: Mixtard, Monotard, Novamix, Actrapid (fast acting)

Tip 1: If the patient is found to be having hypoglycaemia (dangerously low blood sugar), some wards stock Hypostop. This is a paste like substance that the nurse can squirt into the patients mouth and then ask the patient to swallow. This paste (Hypostop) is full of a strong glucose based, fast acting consumable that will rapidly raise the level of glucose within the patient's blood stream.

Tip 2: If there is no Hypostop available, another alternative is to give the patient some tea and a biscuit and maybe put a very small amount of sugar in with the tea. Check with your line manager before doing this.

## Calcichew

### For strong teeth and bones

Calcium is needed for the formation of strong bones and healthy teeth and is involved in helping the blood to clot. This may be given if the patient is found to have low calcium or calcium deficiency.

## Senna (laxative)

### Constipation and bowel evacuation

Senna is a stimulant laxative that can relieve constipation; empty and prepare the bowel for surgery or examination.

## Lactulose (laxative)

### Softens stool. Constipation

Lactulose is a synthetic sugar used to treat constipation. It is broken down in the colon into products that pull water out from the body and into the colon. This water softens stools.

Have you ever wondered what the milky white substance is patients receive when they are fully sedated (put to sleep) for surgery? The substance is called Propofol. Propofol is given via a cannula and will put a patient to sleep within around 20 seconds.

Propofol

## **Sedation**

Anaesthetic and sedation for patients having surgery or are receiving ventilation.

Tip: Many senior nurses have a motto that is: If you do not know what a drug is for, don't give the drug until you do know what the drug is for. Check the BNF if you don't!!

Calpol

## **Pain, temperature**

This medication is for children that are presenting pain and/or temperature. It can be used for children from 2 months to12 years.

Tip: different strengths Calpol works for different aged children
Above, is a list of the most common medications given to patients.

# COMPLAINTS AND PROCEDURES

Everyday people come into hospital presenting a multitude of different medical complaints.  Therefore it is within the nurse's best interest to have a good basic knowledge of common medical procedures and patient complaints.  The next section of this book will concentrate on procedures such as Alzheimer's, Dementia, heart attacks, strokes, head injuries, chest pain, allergic reactions etc.

Go through each section, reading the red title and test yourself on the remaining text. The next section is in alphabetical order.  Mark off the ones that you have learned and continue to revise the remainder.

## Common Medical Complaints

### Abdominal Pain

### Stress, Vomiting, Diarrhoea, Appendix, Gallbladder, Diverticulitis

The patent may be experiencing a dull achy pain to a sharp stabbing sensation in and around the abdomen area. The different areas of pain may can give an indication as to where the problem maybe arising from or what organ maybe causing the pain.

An example of this could be that the patient is experiencing pain from the lower right side of the abdomen.  This indicates that the patient maybe suffering from Appendicitis.  Different areas mean different problems.

Tip 1: Even if you think you know or have a good idea what a problem maybe, be sure not to give you own opinion as the patient may take this as a formal diagnosis.

Many patients look to the nurse for answers as to causes or possible diagnosis of their medical condition.  Make an effort to use the words "possibly", "maybe", "I would rather not say", "you best wait for the doctor to see you". Be clear about your professional boundaries and bear in mind that all of the multidisciplinary team have a different part to play in the rehabilitation of patients.

## Allergic Reaction

## **Hay Fever, Animals, Medications, Food (nuts), materials, bites and stings**

Some indications of an allergic reaction may include; redness or rash, watery eyes, runny nose and sneezing. Some allergic reaction such as anaphylaxis can be more serious and in some cases life threatening. Many mild reactions are treated with anti-histamine medication such a Piriton (Chlorpheniramine).

## Alzheimer's

## **Cause unknown or loss of brain cells**

Alzheimer's is a condition that affects elderly people. Doctors do not know the cause of Alzheimer's and it is quite difficult to diagnose and it affects 5% of people over 65 and 20% of people over 80. The condition is a progressive degenerative disorder and the first symptoms are memory loss followed by the inability to think and understand. For the student nurse and any nurse, this can (in most cases) make your job very challenging. When dealing with patients with Alzheimer's your own tolerance level will be tested from time to time as these people can and will often become very confused and sometimes cannot tell the difference between day and night, whether they are at home or in hospital and in many cases will not co-operate with doctors and nurses. Most patients will die from this condition within 8 years, but some may live with it for up to 20 years.

## Anaemia

## **Internal bleeding, iron, vitamin B12 and folic acid deficiency, cancer**

There are three different types of anaemia: General anaemia, sickle-cell anaemia and haemolytic anaemia. Sickle-cell: this is where the body produces abnormally shaped red blood cells. This disease commonly occurs in people of black origin. Haemolytic anaemia: the red blood cells within the body are being destroyed much quicker than usual. General anaemia: internal bleeding or loss of blood/red blood cells within the body. In mild cases, the patient maybe advised to increase or concentrate on their dietary intake, such as increasing their iron, folic acid and vitamin B12 intake which helps in the production of red blood cells. In more severe cases, the patient may receive iron injections or tablets such as ferrous sulphate.

## Angina

### Clogging of arteries, build up of fatty deposits, oxygen deficiency of the heart

The patient usually feels a sharp stabbing pain around the chest area. In most cases of angina, the pain will diminish or go after around 15 minutes. In many cases of angina, the patient may receive a nitro-glycerine (GTN) spray. This spray opens up and expands the coronary arteries, allowing more oxygen to flow freely to the heart, thus causing the patient less pain.

## Anxiety

### Nerves, worry, stress, tension

Everybody gets anxious from time to time and it is quite normal to have this awareness mechanism within us. Anxiety starts to get out of control when it becomes overwhelming for the patient and they have increased states of panic. Deep expression of fear, sudden outbursts, panic attacks is a few of the factors that outline anxiety.

## Arthritis

### Wear and tear of bones, breakdown of the immune system

The two types of arthritis that you will hear about are: osteoarthritis and rheumatoid arthritis. There is also an inflammatory arthritis and non-inflammatory arthritis.

Osteoarthritis is non-inflammatory (will not inflame) and is very common among older and elderly people and is caused by wear and tear of the bones over a period of time. The symptoms of osteoarthritis include swelling, pain, loss of function in limbs and changes in the joint cartilage. In cases of Osteoarthritis, the doctor may prescribe medication such as Co-codamol and drugs along with opioid based medication such as morphine to deal with what is known as "break through pain".

Rheumatoid arthritis is inflammatory and is cause by a breakdown of the immune system, but is not yet fully understood as to why this occurs. The symptoms of Rheumatoid arthritis are: intense and sudden pain, swelling, redness, warmth and tenderness, loss of motion and function of the joint and joint damage. Of cases of Rheumatoid arthritis, the doctor may prescribe a non-steroidal anti-inflammatory drug (NSAID). This will be a drug that has pain relief and anti-inflammatory properties but no steroids. This maybe a drug such as Ibuprofen or penicillamine.

## Asthma

### Short of breath, Wheezing, panic, coughing

This is a chronic lung condition caused by inflammation and will cause the patient to have recurrent breathing problems and difficulty in breathing (DIB). People with Asthma have extra sensitive airways that are prone to narrowing or obstructing when they become irritated. See inhalers (chapter 1).

## Cancer

### Anxiety, Fear, Lumps

This well known, terrible, and in some cases untreatable disease can come in more than 100 different forms, i.e. skin cancer or brain cancer. The most well known cancer in modern times is breast cancer that affects a large number of women each year and in some cases men are affected by breast cancer too (around 2%).

Cancer is characterised by an uncontrollable growth of malignant (bad) cells that are combined to make up a tumour. These cells invade and destroy surrounding tissue or organs where they can start new cancers if given the opportunity. Early detection of cancer is vital as it can be fatal in some cases.

Cancer can be removed using one or a combination of three methods: chemo therapy (using Cytotoxic Cell killing drugs), radiotherapy (blasting the cancer site with radioactive and killing cells) or surgery. The first two treatments are preferred by many patients as they are less invasive than surgery. A surgery option could be used to cut away and remove the tumour.

## Colic

### Pain, cramps, developing digestive system

This problem occurs in young babies and new born babies. The constant growth of the digestive system causes intermittent pain and cramps. This will cause the baby to cry and may cause stress to the parents. Classic signs of colic are: pulling legs up towards stomach, constant crying, vomiting and diarrhoea and absence of urine.

## Chest Pain

### Pulmonary emboli (Blood clot in artery), angina, heart attack, heart burn, panic attack

Chest pain is probably the most common of all complaints among older people. This does not mean that the complaint exclusively belongs to this group. People of all ages could complain of chest pain due to a multitude of reasons.

A common fear and causes of chest pain is a heart attack. Patients can suffer from mild or severe heart attack depending on the amount of blood and oxygen being restricted to the pathway to the heart. This blockage maybe due to a blood clot within one of the blood vessels surrounding the heart. This will prevent blood from getting to a certain part of the heart muscle and may cause a small section of it to die. This is called an infarct. If this happens or is happening, the patient will experience the above pain due to the infarct around the heart.

The patient maybe experiencing a sharp stabbing pain, crushing sensation, burning or pressure sensation in and around the chest area. As a matter of propriety, the nurse will perform an ECG (electrocardiogram). An ECG records and prints the electrical activity of the heart. The heart uses electrical impulses to create beats and functions. The print out will show an experienced person with ECG skills if there are any abnormalities within the heart. The skilled person or doctor will then make a decision on what course of action to take. The ECG will show if the patient is having a heart attack or any other problems/electrical abnormalities such as AF (Atrial Fibrillation), VF (Ventricular Fibrillation or LAD (Left Access Deviation) for example.

## Diarrhoea and Vomiting

## Infection, bacteria in food poisoning and virus

Diarrhoea and vomiting is caused by infections that lie within the GI (gastrointestinal) tract. This sort of infection could be caused by bacteria on badly prepared food etc. If the problem continues for long periods there is a fear of the person becoming dehydrated. For most health care professionals, the plan will be to make sure that the patient has an adequate fluid intake and rest the digestive system until the bug passes.

## Dementia

## <u>Brain cells are damaged and die faster than usual</u>

Dementia is a condition that affects elderly people.  When older people develop dementia, their brain cells die and become damaged faster than someone without dementia.  This will inevitably affect their interest in activities and memory.  It will also affect their washing, dressing and eating ability and they may eventually lose the ability to look after themselves.  These people need lots of support.

Tip 1: this is an ideal opportunity to get involved with medical and discharge planning as the patient's condition is quite likely to remain stable and this makes it easier to follow and play a key role in their plan.  There are also many numbers of the multidisciplinary team involved in the rehabilitation of elderly patient's so getting involved in this will give you a good insight in to what part the other members play in the rehabilitation process.

Tip 2: Remember that patients with dementia and Alzheimer's can sometimes be very difficult to deal with.  Always remember that you are working as part of a team and are not expected to deal with every situation that is presented to you.  If you feel you are struggling to cope physically and/or mentally, call on your colleagues for help.  You may think that you can struggle and get by, but this will eventually have an effect on your passion for nursing and may change your aspect on patient care in the future.  If you feel that you have had enough and/or are dealing with more than one patient with dementia, remember to take some time out and let someone else take over for a while.

## Diabetes

## <u>Too much or too little insulin in the body, uncontrolled blood sugar</u>

The way in which the body digests food is called metabolism.  After we eat, the food gets broken down into glucose (sugar) and is used for growth and energy. For glucose to get into blood cells, a hormone called insulin must be present. Insulin is produced by a large gland called the pancreas and is located behind the stomach. The pancreas will produce the right amount of insulin after digestion and will move the sugar from the blood in to the cells. In people with diabetes, the pancreas will not operate properly and will produce too little or no insulin. In some cases, the cells will not respond properly to the amount of insulin that is produced and therefore overflowing on to the urine and passed out of the body. This will cause the body to lose its main source of fuel.

In general, diabetes means that the patient has too little or too much sugar within their blood stream. The condition where there is a patient presenting with high volume of sugar in their blood is known as hyperglycaemia or hyperglycaemic and a patient presenting with too little insulin in the blood stream is known as a hypoglycaemia or hypoglycaemic. Blood sugar should be around 4 to 6 mmols (mmols is the amount that blood sugar is measured in). Some patient's blood sugar is naturally higher and therefore that figure will be normal for them. There are two different types of diabetes.

Type 1 Diabetes : This is where the patient will be given a regular dose of insulin via a needle or insulin pen (insulin controlled)
Type 2 Diabetes : Patient will use tablets or food to control the amount of insulin that is being produced by the pancreas or their blood sugar levels.

Tip 1: with type 1 diabetes, think of the "1" being the needle or representing the needle. This will give an indication that the patient is receiving insulin and you will not get confused as to whether it is type 1 or 2 that you give the patient insulin.

Tip 2: in hand, over or report, the nurse handing over may refer to the patient as NIDDM or IDDM. NIDDM stands for "non insulin dependent diabetic mellitus" and IDDM stands for "insulin dependent diabetic mellitus". You may be wondering what the mellitus part is about. There are two overall types of diabetes that being: Diabetes mellitus and Diabetes insipidus (caused by the inability of the kidneys to conserve water). I will not go into detail about Diabetes insipudus as you will very rarely or will never come across this complaint or condition within your nursing career.

Tip 3, if you spot any unusual behaviour from patient or if they seem weak, disorientated or confused, carry out a full set of observations (blood pressure, temperature, respirations and pulse). Also, check their fluid i ntake (low fluid intake can cause confusion and UTI's-urinary tract infections) as well as the patient's blood sugar. Talking and communication with the patient is always a good indicator as to whether something is wrong. In most cases, it will be one of these three actions that will produce an abnormal reading. Gather all of your readings and confer your findings with the nurse in charge who will help you determine the right course of action to take. You should be praised for being thorough!

## Emphysema

### Shortness of breath, difficulty in breathing, low sats

This lung condition is caused when the alveoli (air sacs within the lung) are damaged and no longer function properly. The patient will not be able to breathe to full capacity and will clearly show signs of difficulty in breathing. This condition can in some cases be fatal.

## Fracture (cracked or broken bone)

### Accident, falling, assault, fragile bones

There are two main types of fracture that can occur. These are: open and closed fracture. A closed fracture means that the bone has not penetrated or protruded through the skin, therefore the bone will not be visible but will be broken.

An open fracture means that the bone is clearly visible protruding through the skin. Other factors depend on the type of fracture. There are a number of different ways a bone can be broken:

A patient with a fractured bone could present the following: abnormal or bent limbs, redness or/and swelling, bruising, or be clammy and sweaty.

The two main factors associated with a fracture are pain and bleeding. The patient may be given a drug called Entonox (usually given in A&E Accident & Emergency) and Maternity. Entonox is given to patients as a gas that can be self administered and breathed in. Patients are given a mouth piece and are asked to take as much or as little as they need, depending on the amount of pain experienced and their pain threshold. This gas is very fast acting and has a very short half life (time of action till the time the action starts to decline).

Orthopaedic stands for the study of bones. In general, anything to do with bones will come under the orthopaedic part of your profession.

Tip 1: sometimes nurses and doctors refer to a certain group of people called "orthopod/s" this is hospital slang and is used to identify a doctor or a group of doctors responsible for looking after people with bone complaints or conditions. These doctors are also known as orthopaedic (bone) doctor/s or the orthopaedic team.

Tip 2: You may also hear the word "max fax", this stands for Maxilla Facial. This is the upper part of the jaw that is located above the mandible. There are a certain group of doctors that specialises in dealing with this part of the face.

## Hepatitis

## Inflammation of the liver, flu like symptoms, fever, jaundice, dark urine

This is a chronic condition of the liver that results in inflammation (swelling) caused by a number of reasons. Some of the reasons could include: viral and bacterial infections, trauma, alcoholism or drug reactions. There are different strains of the disease. Strain B and C being most common. A national vaccination programme has been in place for many years to prevent the spread of Hepatitis. All health care personnel that come into contact with patients should be up-to-date with the hepatitis immunisation. If in doubt, contact your line manager or mentor who will tell you to contact occupational health. Being up to date is a must as you will regularly come across patients with the disease!

Tip 1: itis is Latin for inflammation. Hepatic = liver and itis = inflammation. Therefore Hepatitis = inflammation of the liver. Inflammation of the tonsil = tonsillitis. Get it!

Tip 2: many medical terms derive from the Latin language due to medical science first being written in Latin.

## High Blood Pressure (hypertension)

### Smoking, drinking, bad dietary intake, hereditary

Hypertension is one of the most common chronic diseases amongst older people (long duration). A patient can experience high blood pressure (Hypertension) and low blood pressure (hypotension).

Hypertension can also be caused by medication problems elsewhere within the body. This type of complaint is called secondary hypertension. Hypertension means the build-up of pressure within the arteries. Being overweight can increase the risk of hypertension. Running, walking, swimming, cycling and regular exercise can prevent or reduce the risk of hypertension.

Stopping smoking reducing the amount of alcohol consumption and a good dietary intake is strongly recommended for patients suffering from this condition. Patients may be given medication such an Amlodipine to open the arteries and lower their blood pressure.

# Pyrexia (high temperature)

## Infection, drugs, malignancy, endocrine

High temperature can be caused by many different aspects and the most likely cause is infection somewhere within the body. Whatever the cause the temperature must be controlled. If you come across a patient that is presenting with a high temperature it is recommended that the patient removes some clothing, recommend a fan and/or open a window where possible. If you do not see a drop in temperature check on the prescription chart to see if the patient has been prescribed Paracetamol. This is usually the first port of call with regard to using medication. Paracetamol is one of the very few medications that can be written on the medication chart as what's known as a STAT (once only) dose medication by a qualified nurse (Not student, unless authorised, supervised and countersigned by a qualified member of staff).

Tip 1: check for allergies. The patient may be allergic to Paracetamol also check to ensure patient does not have any underlying liver problems.

Tip 2: a slight temperature is commonly known as a "low grade pyrexia", this maybe a temperature of around 37.2. Anything higher maybe considered a temperature or pyrexia and a course of action should be taken. A temperature of 40.0 or more is considered to be hyperpyrexia and an immediate course of action should be taken to lower the temperature and to ensure it does not climb any higher. This should be given your full attention as the patients' temperature is at a very dangerous level.

## Hypothyroidism

## Under active thyroid, thyroid hormone deficiency

This occurs when the immune system attacks the thyroid tissue with white blood cells and antibodies due to the body recognising the tissue as a foreign body. Thus, the thyroid gland may become swollen and enlarged, this is called a goitre.  An under active thyroid may also develop after patients have had thyroid surgery or radioactive therapy.Sometime children are born without a thyroid gland or with a thyroid that does not function properly.  Some of the symptoms of hypothyroidism include:  depression,  constipation,  weight  gain, feeling cold and fatigue. A blood sample will be taken from the patient and results should determine thyroid complications.  Many patients receive a diagnosis of an under active thyroid and will receive a medication called Thyroxine.  In most cases, this medication will be taken for the rest of their lives.

## Jaundice

## **Bilirubin in the blood, Hepatitis A, infection from food, alcohol and drug abuse**

A patient with jaundice can easily be spotted due to the yellow tinge in the whites of the eyes and on the surface of the skin.  The liver would normally excreted bilirubin and other waste products from the patients are unable to be excreted and therefore build up in the body, presenting the patient with a yellow tinge that is commonly known as jaundice.

Treatment for this depends on what may be causing the problem with the liver and will also depend on the diagnosis from the doctor.

## MRSA (multi resistant staphylococcus aureus)

## **Bug resistant to most or all antibiotics**

It is most likely that you would have heard of this in the news or media. This is the most common of all bugs that is resistant to most antibiotics. In many cases this infection is acquired within the hospital (Nosocomial) and is sometimes caused by poor hand washing and infection control.  It can be passed on skin to skin contact as nurses go from patient to patient. Patients with open or post operative wounds are more at risk.  This is because MRSA causes many complications such as prevention or prolonged wound healing. Wounds may not heal when MRSA is present or may take excessive amounts of time to heal. This will cause many implications when you are presented with a patient with pressure ulcers and MRSA. This is sometimes known as a staph (Staphylococcal) infection. Patients with MRSA should be treated with caution and gloves and apron must be worn when dealing or coming into contact with these patients.

These patients will be barrier nursed and should be quarantined off from other patients due to the risk of infection. If there is room available, patients with MRSA will be in a side room with a barrier nursing sign by the door. Nurses should apply gloves and aprons before entering the room and remove gloves and aprons and wash hands before exiting the room. As an extra precaution all medical professional are advised to rub alcohol gel into their hands after dealing with patients with MRSA.

Tip: throughout your shift, your arms are the least protected area of your body. Make it a habit to rub alcohol gel on these areas too.

## Pressure Ulcer (pressure sore/bed sore)

## <u>Restricted movement, lack of blood and oxygen to body, vulnerable parts of the body</u>

This is another very common sight within the hospital and can occur in people of all ages from children to adults. Pressure ulcers will occur in patients that sit or lie in one place for too long or are unable or have unrestricted movement in bed. With elderly patients, the problem is more widespread due to reluctance to move and may result in being a heavier work load for the nurse. Patients that have minimal or restricted mobility should be encouraged and helped to move or turn every 20 minutes to 2 hours (depending on ability to move).

There are some areas that are more prone to pressure ulcers than others. These are the mainly the bony parts of the body where there is little flesh between the bone and the outside hard surface, thus restricting the amount of oxygen and blood flow to that part of the body.

Good nutrition is also very important when it comes to preventing and curing pressure ulcers. Poor nutrition does not cause pressure ulcers, but makes it difficult for them heal and makes it easier for them to start. Always encourage good food and fluid intake with your patients and regularly check for pressure ulcers. If a patient has a pressure ulcer, it must be re-dressed on a regular basis and regularly monitored for them to progressively heal.

Tip 1: as and when you wash or bed bath patients, kill two birds with one stone and at the same time check for any pressure ulcers or red areas that may have developed (Especially around the sacral area and heels).

Tip 2: pressure ulcers can sometimes be a likely breeding ground for MRSA so regular checks to make sure that MRSA is not present is always a good thing.

## Stroke/Cerebral Vascular Accident (CVA)

## **Blocked blood vessels in the brain, ruptured blood vessels in the brain**

A stroke occurs when the blood flow to the brain stops. This is due to two reasons:

Ischemic stroke is the more common of the two. This is where the patient develops a blood clot that blocks an artery or vessel responsible for transporting blood to the brain.

Haemorrhagic stroke occurs when a vessel supplying blood to the brain ruptures and leaks blood in to the brain tissue.

Both of the above will cause brain cells to die and the patient will quickly start to develop symptoms of left or right sided weakness with their legs, arms and face. Confusion and difficulty in speaking, poor coordination and headache may occur.

Patients may be on medication to break up the clots that lie within the brain. Intense rehabilitation to restore activities of daily living will be a priority.

TIA or Transient Ischemic Attack is the result of a small temporary interruption of the supply of blood to the brain due to a blockage or rupture in a vessel. These are sometimes referred to as mini stokes. Most patients recover from these types of attack but the rehabilitation process can be variable.

## Urinary Tract Infection (UTI)

## **Bacteria, bad hygiene, sexually transmitted**

Most nurses and other health care professionals will refer to this as a UTI and is a very common site within hospitals and especially with elderly patients. Bacteria (also known as BUGS) enter the body (usually) via the urethra, (the tube from the bladder to where urine exits the body being the vagina or penis) it then enters and stays within the bladder and the urinary tract. The cause of a UTI is usually bad hygiene, lack of catheter cleaning or poor management. This infection (in most cases) causes moderate to severe pain for the patient and can also make the patient confused. In most or all cases UTI's can be cured with a simple course of oral or IV antibiotics (see Antibiotics).

An indication of a UTI might be dark cloudy or smelly urine, pain when passing urine, urine retention (unable to pass urine), frequent or urgent urination and sometimes asymptomatic (no signs or symptoms at all). If any of these elements are present, you will need to perform a dip-stick urine test to test for any abnormalities. You can use your own initiative to perform a dip-stick urine test. You will first need a sample of urine, there are two different ways of obtaining urine, these are MSU and CSU.

**CSU**: Catheter Stream Urine (obtaining a sample of urine from the catheter). For this procedure you will need a cardboard tray, a ten ml (millilitre) syringe, streret or pre-injection swab (small pad soaked with isopropyl alcohol used for cleaning) green needle and a urine sample bottle.

When you have gathered all these items, see your mentor or line manager who will show you the process of obtaining a sample of urine.

**MSU**: Mid Stream Urine asking the patient to wee into a pot!

Tip: if you can, ask the patient to discard the first part of the wee, as this may be contaminated with outside elements.

When you have a sample, you are now ready to dip-stick the urine, using a dip-stick strip test or urinalysis machine test (clinitec)

Show your finds to your mentor, the doctor, or the nurse in charge, who might ask you to send a sample to the laboratory for further, more accurate or wider testing of your sample. For this, you will need to fill out a microbiology form that will go with your sample in a clear bag to the laboratory.

# ESSENTIAL ANATOMY AND PHYSIOLOGY

In this section you will be shown the purpose and primary function of all the main organs within the human body. To have a good knowledge of just the basic function provides you with a mini mental map which will enable you to confidently locate the area of each organ, explaining its basis function. This knowledge is very rarely learned by student nurses, but I personally feel that a good knowledge of this is one of the essential building blocks to becoming a great nurse. Again, this section will be explained by giving the name of the organ first, then the basis function, then a small explanation about the organ. Remember that only a number of basic organs will be touched upon and only the basic functions will be explained.

Lets go!

## The Brain

## <u>Thought, all bodily function, memory, self awareness</u>

The brain and spinal cord combined make up the central nervous system. The rest of the nerves that are connected to the brain and spinal cord are called the peripheral nerves. The brain makes up around 2% of the human body weight and use 20% of the blood flow and takes up around 20% of the bodies oxygen supply. The brain holds within it, two very important glands. The pituitary gland and hypothalamus.

The pituitary gland is responsible for producing ADH (Ant diuretic hormones). This increases the amount of absorption in the bloodstream by the kidneys. Oxytocin stimulates milk production after child birth and contract the uterus during childbirth. Melanocyte controls skin pigmentation. Luteinizing hormone and follicle stimulating hormones stimulates the testis or ovaries. Thyroid-stimulating hormone stimulates the thyroid gland. Adrenocorticotropic hormone stimulates the adrenal glands, stimulated growth hormone. Prolactin stimulates milk production after giving birth.

The hypothalamus gland is responsible for body weight, fluid and electrolyte balance, body temperature and blood pressure.

The brain also has another very important part to it called the medulla oblongata. It is located at the lower part of the brainstem and is responsible for relaying nerve signals between the brain and spinal cord and controlling our autonomic functions.

Common problems of the brain could include stroke/cerebral vascular accident (CVA) or mini stroke/TIA (Transient Ischemic Attack)

## The Heart

## **Pumping blood around the body for the transport of oxygen and nutrients**

The heart is the primary part of the cardiovascular system (blood tubes within the body). It is primary function is to pump blood around the body.

The heart uses electrical impulse to beat and makes use of its four chambers to collect in de-oxygenated (used) blood from veins/tissues around the body, then sends that blood to the lungs to collect oxygen, then goes back to the heart and is then pumped to all other parts of the body whilst transporting much needed oxygen and nutrients.

The heart is around the size and weight of your fist. It is one of the most important parts of the human anatomy but also one of the most abused due to smoking, drinking and maintaining a poor diet. Common problems of the heart include: Myocardial Infarction (MI) commonly known as a heart attack.

## The Lungs

### Breathing, expelling carbon dioxide, gaseous exchange

The lungs are the main part of the respiratory system. When we breathe, air travels down the trachea (wind pipe) and in to the lungs. The lungs are filled with around 6 million tiny little air pockets called Alveoli. These alveoli will allow air to filter through and pass into the blood stream. The body will then extract the oxygen it needs from the inhaled air and will discard the rest (carbon dioxide) through the same route (out through the lungs and the mouth). A substance within red cells called haemoglobin carries the oxygen we receive to all parts of the body.

Common problems with the lungs: Emphysema and Asthma.

## The Liver

### Breaks down fats, produces urea, storage of vitamins and minerals, cholesterol production

The liver is the largest gland in the human body and weighs around ¾ pounds. It produces special bile and that converts glucose into glycogen. The urea produces and makes up the main substance of urine. The liver also makes up the building blocks of protein that are called amino acids and responsible for storing vitamins A, D, K and B12 and to maintain the appropriate level of glucose in the blood.

Two main diseases of the liver include: Hepatitis and cancer. See chapter 2.

## Kidneys

### Filter and remove metabolic waste products from the blood

The human kidneys are located inside of the lower back and are shaped similar to two larges beans. They are used to filter, clean and remove waste products from the blood and excreting/discarding it as urine.  They also maintain the amount of chemicals in the blood (homeo-stasis) such as sodium, potassium and phosphate.

Problems with kidneys : possible problems with kidneys include nephritis and nephropathy.  These problems among others can cause kidney failure and may result in the patient having dialysis whereby an artificial kidney is used to dialysis a patient on a dialysis machine around 3 times per week. This is also known as renal dialysis.

## Pancreas

## Production of juices to help digest food, production of insulin

The pancreas is part of the endocrine and exocrine system and is located just behind the stomach and is around 15cm in length (around the size of your hand).  Its main function is to produce pancreatic juices or enzymes to help in the process of braking down food.  The other main task of the pancreas is to produce insulin to control the sugar levels within the body.

Common problems with the pancreas: diabetes and cancer.  See chapter 2.

## Gall Bladder

## Produces bile for fat digestion

When food containing fats is digested, the gall bladder released bile to help in the digestion of such fats.  This bile has been previously received from the liver, but has been stored in the gall bladder, ready to be released when fats are detected.

Common problems with the gall bladder : gall stones and infection.
Gall stones can be associated with a bad dietary intake.  It is possible for the gall bladder to be removed and for the body to still function like normal.

# Appendix

## **Purpose unknown/unclear**

This organ is a worm like shape that hangs near to the small and large intestine. It does not serve us with any real function, but does contain some lymphoid tissue (cells that are able to produce antibodies to fight infection).

Problems with the human appendix can include appendicitis. This can be treated with antibiotics or in severe cases can be removed with surgery. This removal leaves scar just above the groin area. It is a common procedure and you may well have seen this scar before. The body does not need this organ to function.

Tip 1: by this stage of the book, you should know what an appendicitis is! Remember "itis" = Latin for inflammation.

## Intestine

## **Digestion, Absorption of water, excretion of faeces**

The human intestine is split up into two parts and has different functions. The small intestine is used for absorbing most foods. The large intestine is used for extracting water and will then make faeces from human waste products. The small intestine consists of the Jejunum and Ileum. The large intestine consists of the ascending colon, transverse colon and descending colon.

Common problems with the intestines: parasites/worms and pancreatitis = inflammation of the pancreas
Remember "itis" = Latin for inflammation

## Bladder

### **Storing Urine**

This is a simple organ used for storing urine that has been received from the kidneys and will pass such urine whenever we feel the need!
Common problems with bladder: cancer of the bladder.

## Bowel

### **Absorbs nutrients, Secretes waste as faeces**

This bowel absorbs most of the nutrients from the food and drink that we consume. It will then excrete waste products via the back passage as stool/faeces. There are two parts to the bowel being the small bowel and the large bowel. The large bowel can be split up in to three/four sections, Ascending colon, Transverse colon, Descending colon and Rectum. These sections absorb fluid from food. The small bowel breaks food down and absorbs vital nutrients.

Problems with the bowel: Irritable Bowel Syndrome (IBS), constipation, bowel cancer.

## Spleen

### **Storing blood components, blood management, producing antibodies**

The spleen is a small organ around the size of your fist, and is located to the left of the abdomen. It is used to store certain blood components such as platelets. It also cleans the blood, removing any damaged or old worn out blood cells and removing any other particles found. It is also used to regulate blood flow to the liver and produces a special type of white blood cells called Lymphocytes (antibodies).

Problems with the spleen may include enlargement, sometimes due to infection or disease of the liver.

# ABBREVATIONS

During your work as a student nurse and as a staff nurse, you will very frequently come across abbreviations. Abbreviations are very widespread and are commonly used on the wards by all members of the multidisciplinary team. Some of these abbreviations will be common and easily understood and some will not. A list of the most common abbreviations you will come across immediately whilst working on the wards and departments are listed below.

Feel free to use abbreviations yourself but keep in mind that they must be official to the hospital you are working in at the time.

## Staff Abbreviations

RGN     Registered General Nurse

RNA     Registered Nurse Adult

RSCN    Registered Sick Children's Nurse

RMN     Registered Mental Nurse/Psychiatric Nurse

FY1     Foundation year 1

FY2     Foundation year 2

CMT     Core Medical Trainer (on way to be registrar)

REG     Registrar

CONS    Consultant

HCA     Health Care Assistant

ST/N    Student Nurse

S/N     Staff Nurse

C/N     Charge Nurse

S/R     Sister

SSR     Senior Sister (formerly Ward Manager)

## General Abbreviations

MSU     Mid Stream Urine

CSU     Catheter Stream Urine

BO      Bowels Open

D & V   Diarrhoea and vomiting

C DIFF  Clostridium Difficile

IDC     In-dwelling Catheter

TWOC    Trial without Catheter

NBM     Nil By Mouth

SOB     Shortness of Breath

DIB     Difficulty in Breathing

BP      Blood Pressure

TEMP    Temperature

RESP    Respiration

HR      Heart Rate

| | |
|---|---|
| SATS | Oxygen Saturation/Oximetry |
| TPR | Temperature, Pulse, Respiration |
| COPD | Chronic Obstructive Pulmonary Disease |
| TB | Tuberculosis |
| PE | Pulmonary Embolism |
| CA | Cancer |
| METS | Metastasis |
| CVA | Cerebral Vascular Accident |
| TIA | Transient Ischemic Attack |
| CCF | Congestive Cardiac Failure |
| AF | Ventricular Fibrillation |
| ARF | Acute Renal Failure |
| CRF | Chronic Renal Failure |
| FFP | Fresh Frozen Plasma |
| IDDM | Insulin Dependent Diabetes Mellitus |
| NIDDM | Non-Insulin Dependent Diabetes Mellitus |
| DM | Diabetes Mellitus |
| DVT | Deep Vein Thrombosis |
| UTI | Urinary Tract Infection |

CXR    Chest X Ray

AXR    Abdominal X Ray

MRI    Magnetic Resonance Imaging

CT     Computer Tomography

ECG    Electrocardiogram

NG     Naso Gastric tube

RX     Prescriptive Treatment

ABG    Arterial Blood Gases

MRSA   Multi/Methicillin Resistant Staphylococcus Aurous

OTT    Out to Toilet

BIPAP  Biphasic Positive Airway Pressure

OBS    Observations

## Medication/Drug Chart Abbreviations

OD     Once Daily

BD     Twice Daily

TDS    Three Times Daily

QDS    Four Times Daily

PRN    Pro Re Nata (as and when required)

STAT   Statum (One off initial dose)

TTA     Tablets to take away

MCG     Microgram (1000 Microgram = 1 Milligram)

G       Gram (1 Gram = 1000 Milligram)

KG      Kilogram (1 Kilogram = 1000 Grams)

# ADMINISTRATIONS ROUTE

The route of administration will tell you the way/s in which a drug should be given to the patient. Such routes are usually abbreviated on the drug chart or in the patient's notes.

Tip 1: remember that anything IM or IV should be checked by two qualified/qualified and student nurses before being given to the patient.

Tip 2: if you are unsure **_DO NOT DO IT_**. Do not ever assume that something should be done in a certain way. If you are unclear or unsure of how to do something STOP and seek advice from your mentor or line manager who will give you guidance and advice. Even if your mentor is unavailable at the time, feel free to ask any qualified nurse that is on duty.

NEB/S  Nebulisers

PO     Per OS (by mouth/Oral)

SL     Sublingually (under the tongue)

PR     Per Rectum (back passage)

PV     Per Vagina (via the vagina)

IV     Intravenously (in the vein)

IM     Intramuscularly (in the muscle)

SC     Subcutaneously (under the subcutaneous layer of the skin)

TOP    Topical

INH    Inhaler

# COMMUNICATION

You may have had the experience of asking a question to another member of the MDT and receiving a short, sharp and discrete answer, an explanation that takes too long, a defensive or slightly aggressive answer or you may have been ignored altogether.

This happens from time to time due to the fact that you are working with all kinds of different people that have individual personalities.

We may be looking after the same person/patient but underneath we are all different and may respond in different ways. If you get an unusual, un-expected or abrupt answer, try not to retaliate or rise to it. Maintain your professionalism and always give answers to the best of your knowledge and ability.

Try not to bluff your way out a question, if you do not know, just say so and state that you will find out and come back to them. This also ensures you are able give a better response next time to the same or similar question is presented to you. As a student, you are not expected to know everything, but as your confidence grows, you will start to remember more and more about your patients and you will naturally have a broader and clearer overview of your management area/patients.

If you are polite in your responses, you may NOT always see the respect you gained by doing this straight away. It may be some months down the line until you start to hear good feedback about yourself from increasing numbers of the MDT. This will give you an enormous boost of enthusiasm and confidence and will remind you of the benefits of good communica-tion. Nursing is a stressful area of work however you look at it, but its how you deal with this stress that makes you a good or great nurse. The best nurses are the ones that are able to maintain a good stable line of commu-nication. Even if it is hectic on the ward floor and there is not enough time to do everything, they are still able to communicate to people with a polite manner and give a clear and concise response.

Sometimes this does not come naturally to people, but is a skill that needs to be nurtured and will come automatically in time as you progress in your nursing career. Do the best you can and keep in mind that it may seem from time to time that your best may sometimes not be enough. Do not take it personally, that's nursing and all part of the job.

Feel free to use abbreviations as this will take up less space on your hand over sheets. It may be an idea to have a black pen as well as a red pen when taking hand over. The black pen can be used to write down general details being given by the nurse doing the hand over, whereas as red pen can be used to make a note of things such as infections, important jobs and areas of high risk.

Remember that the only silly question is the question you didn't ask!!

Ask as many questions as you need to during hand over. Other members of the team should be pleased that you are eager to get things right as well as showing a good degree of assertiveness too. Add on to your hand over sheet as you work through your shift as you may need this if you are asked to hand your patients back over to the incoming shift/team.

Good communication as well as good bedside maner will be an essential part of your entire career and although it will not always be possible to please your patients all of the time, however to have a good bedside manner with your patients as well as their families will help you a great deal in the way of building rapport and trust. If you have trust with your patients then you will find that they will also help you to help them and in turn will make your job much easier and so much more rewarding too.

After report/hand over, make a point of going round and saying hello to all of your patients. This again helps to build up trust and will also let you know immediately if anything is not how it should be. As a student nurse, you now have a P.I.N. (Professional identification number) and will be registered as a student nurse with the NMC. As this is the case you are now deemed responsible and partly/jointly account-able to the patients you are allocated, so with this in mind you should want to know what is going on straight after hand over.

Ask your patients if they're ok and do a quick visual check to ensure things like wrist bands are on, bedside dry wipe boards have the correct infor-mation on them, catheters that need emptying etc. Remember that HCA's (Health Care Assistants) are there to help and assist you as they also will be when you become a staff nurse so do your best to get them on your side as a good HCA is priceless!

Patient families can sometimes be the most challenging part of caring for someone. Again, do your best to get then on your side. Rather than talk from the end of the bed, pull up a chair and sit among the family. This sometimes goes a long way whilst trying to build up a bit of trust. Not all nurses are good at communicating like this so if you can get good at it then it may give you the opportunity to be able to instil a lot of trust early on with your patients and their families.

If a family asks you a question about their relative and you don't know or you're not sure, then don't be afraid to say so. They would much rather your honesty and that you get back to them with the correct information when you are able to find this out.

# PATIENT COMMUNICATION

Good patient communication is a large part of nursing and should also go hand in hand with communication with relatives.

The NMC's Code of Professional Conduct, Clause 3.1, states that all patients and clients have the right to receive information about their condition and Clause 2.4 of the Code also states the relevance in helping individuals gain access to information relevant to them. This basically means that (you) the nurse should do your best to keep patient and relatives up to date in what is going on. They will feel more at ease; the more they are kept up to date of their current situation.

When doing this, one needs to use a certain amount of rationale. Keep the patient informed with things like test times and dates, estimated time of discharge and medical plans, but do not inform the patient as to the results of CT scans, biopsy results etc. This is the job of the doctor and you should urge the patient to wait until seeing the doctor to obtain these results.

Treat each patient as an individual! After dealing with one patient, make an effort to take a fresh approach to the next. Patients need you to give a certain amount of empathy (putting yourself in their shoes) when communicating to them.

If you are allocated patients to look after during your shift, it will be down to you to communicate between the MDT and the patient. Do not be put out by this, thinking that you are now under a great amount of pressure. Be professional in your approach and realise that the more you know about your patient, the easier it will be to communicate about them.

Before each nursing placement shift (on arrival), you will be invited in to report or handover. This is an opportunity for all members of nursing staff to communicate and inform the next nursing shift what has been going on with each patient. Handover will last for approximately 15 - 30 minutes, depending on speciality of ward. Most wards also give a walk about handover. This allows the nurse a more personal report and a good opportunity to put a face to the name.

You should have pens and paper at the ready. During handover and especially if you think you are going to be allocated a patient to look after. You will need to be ready to write down as much information as you can about each patient.

As a student nurse, you may feel like you're a staff nurse already from time to time, however never be tempted to cross the line with your responsibilities and boundaries. There will be plenty of time after you qualify to change IV fluids, give injections and be in charge, so with this in mind use your time as a student nurse to refine your basic nursing skills as your patients will benefit from a holistic/hands on approach in a big way. You should be working as supernumerary (In addition to normal staff numbers) and therefore will leave you with plenty of time to complete skills books, reflect with your mentor and develop your overall skills as a future qualified nurse.

Brilliant bedside maner and good hands on nursing skills is not as common place as it was in past years so your time as a student will give you a chance to make these skills a natural part of who you are and what you do even without thinking about it after you qualify. Make sure you enjoy your time as a student and have fun as three years will go by much quicker than you think!

INDEX

**Airway,** 16, 17, 29, 52
Allergic Reaction, 26, 27, 29
Antibiotics, 20
arthritis, 12, 31
Asthma, 19, 31, 32, 47
**Bacteria infections**, 22
Bladder, 48, 49
blood, 12
**blood pressure**, 16, 17, 36, 38, 39, 46
Bowel, 50
brain, 12, 29, 32, 33, 34, 42, 43, 45, 46
**Breathing**, 18, 19, 20, 46, 52
**Breathing and airway**, 19
Co-codamol, 10
Co-Codamol, 10
**complaints and procedures**, 27
**controlled drug**, 14
Dementia, 27, 34
Diabetes, 34, 35, 36, 53
drug/prescription, 11
**Fights bacteria,** 22
fracture, 36, 37
**Heart**, 15
Hepatitis, 37, 38, 40, 47
**high temperature**, 10, 11, 39
Ibuprofen, 12, 31
**impulsive behaviour.,** 18
**inflammation**, 10, 11, 12, 32, 38, 49
injected intravenously, 14
**Internal**, 30
kidneys, 22, 36, 45, 47, 48, 49
**Kills bacteria**, 21
laxatives, 9, 26
**Medical complaints and procedures**, 27
Medication/drug chart, 54

**Moderate to severe pain.,** 13
muscular, 10
**Nausea and Vomiting**, 15
Nebulizer, 19
overdose, 11
Pain relief, 10
paracetamol, 10, 11
**Stress,,** 28
Stroke, 42
Tablet or injection, 12
Temperature, 52
tenderness,, 12
Urine, 44, 49, 52
vitamins, 47

Made in the USA
Columbia, SC
19 June 2017